Real

646.
7242

s

## REAL LIFE GUIDES

Practical guides for practical people

In this increasingly sophisticated world the need for manually skilled people to build our homes, cut our hair, fix our boilers and make our cars go is greater than ever. As things progress, so the level of training and competence required of our skilled manual workers increases.

In this new series of career guides from Trotman, we look in detail at what it takes to train for, get into and be successful at a wide spectrum of practical careers. *Real Life Guides* aim to inform and inspire young people and adults alike by providing comprehensive yet hard-hitting and often blunt information about what it takes to succeed in these careers.

The other titles in the series are:

*Real Life Guide: the Armed Forces*

*Real Life Guide: Carpentry & Cabinet-Making*

*Real Life Guide: Catering*

*Real Life Guide: Construction*

*Real Life Guide: Electrician*

*Real Life Guide: Hairdressing*

*Real Life Guide: Plumbing*

*Real Life Guide: the Motor Industry*

*Real Life Guide: Retailing*

*Real Life Guide: Working Outdoors*

trotman

*Real
Life*

**GUIDES**

CRAVEN COLLEGE

THE BEAUTY
INDUSTRY

Samantha Taylor

*Real Life Guide to the Beauty Industry*
This first edition published in 2004 by Trotman and Company Ltd
2 The Green, Richmond, Surrey TW9 1PL

© Trotman and Company Limited 2004

**Editorial and Publishing Team**
**Author** Samantha Taylor
**Editorial** Mina Patria, Editorial Director; Rachel Lockhart,
Commissioning Editor; Anya Wilson, Editor; Bianca Knights,
Assistant Editor
**Production** Ken Ruskin, Head of Pre-press and Production
**Sales and Marketing** Deborah Jones, Head of Sales and
Marketing
**Advertising** Tom Lee, Commercial Director
**Managing Director** Toby Trotman

**Designed by XAB**

British Library Cataloguing in Publication Data
A catalogue record for this book is available from the British
Library

ISBN  0 85660 996 X

Typeset by Photoprint, Torquay
Printed and bound in Great Britain by Cromwell Press,
Trowbridge, Wiltshire

# Real Life

*Real Life*

## GUIDES

## CONTENTS

# Acknowledgements

I would like to thank the many people who gave up their time to answer my questions – especially Tiffany Tarrant at Habia.

As always, thanks to Pete for his amazing patience (most of the time) when sorting out our girls whilst I was stuck to the computer in a race against time!

# About the author

Samantha Taylor has 21 years' experience in the beauty industry and has taught for 18 years covering Health and Beauty, Key and Basic Skills as an Assessor and Verifier.

She has written a book on the new standards and qualification in Beauty at S/NVQ Level 1 and has piloted a work-related learning scheme in Beauty for school students, working as both course designer and tutor. She has also jointly developed Connect2Beauty, an online learning facility that offers NVQs in Beauty Therapy that are fully approved and accredited by Edexcel.

# Introduction

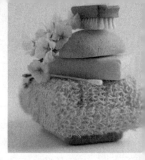

A career in beauty therapy offers many different opportunities. You can do something you love, have fun, meet exciting people and even get the chance to travel, all whilst helping others feel good about themselves. From working in a salon, being your own boss, to cruising the seas – beauty can offer you all this and the chance to progress to management level with a top salary to match!

As the health and beauty industry is one of the fastest-growing sectors in the UK, there is great demand for quality staff with excellent communication skills and commitment to the job. Exciting opportunities with good financial rewards in a flexible and fun environment are there for the right person.

Employment opportunities can range from working in health spas, hospitals and prisons to being a make-up artist on photographic shoots. You may eventually wish to share your knowledge and skills as an educator in a college or work on a beauty magazine as a writer. High demand for beauty therapists means that there is a vast range of opportunities within the industry and, although salaries can be low at the start, the chance to earn excellent wages is there for the right people.

Beauty therapy is a career that you can take with you, wherever your personal life leads you. There will always be someone who will want his or her legs waxed, feet pedicured and achy back massaged. It is no longer a luxury to have these treatments – they are all part of a busy person's lifestyle and maintenance. If you are first-rate at what you do, you will never be short of work.

## DID YOU KNOW?

There are approximately 30,000 vacancies in the UK hair and beauty industry because of a national recruitment shortage of qualified and skilled staff.

Beauty therapy is not restrictive and gains strength from the wide range of talents, personalities, nationalities, abilities and ages that qualify. Although beauty salons can claim exemption from the Sex Discrimination Act and the vast majority of beauty and holistic therapists are female, the number of male therapists is rising – especially as it becomes more acceptable for men to take an interest in beauty treatments too!

In order to make informed decisions about a career in beauty you need to be able to find good-quality and accurate information about the industry – about the types of career options open to you, what you should expect to give to your career and what you can expect to get out of it, and the sources of education and training that can help you get on. This guide is for anyone wanting to train, currently training or who is already qualified and wants to progress further. It details everything you need to know to help you make the right decisions. At the end of the book is a useful list of resources, which help you take your research further.

# Job profiles

Mention the beauty industry and most people will immediately think of a beauty salon, probably much like the one (combined with a hairdressing salon) featured in Channel 4's *The Salon* (although this is not a true represention of the industry and its high standards.) They will think of manicures, pedicures, facials and body waxing and perhaps of more unusual treatments such as hydrotherapy (water-based treatments) and reflexology (holistic foot message). The salon – and to a lesser extent the spa – certainly does form the heart and hub of the beauty profession, but there is a great deal more variety in the industry – both in terms of the range of jobs available and the location where these jobs are carried out, be it a cruise ship, hospital or department store.

In this chapter, we'll look at the full range of jobs available – the type of work they involve, the training they require, the pay and hours and what you can do now to get yourself into that particular area. On page 4, there's a diagram that will give you an overview of the opportunities available.

In every job, you cannot replace high-quality training on your path to success. The most widely recognised beauty-industry qualifications are known as National Vocational Qualifications (NVQs) or, in Scotland, the Scottish Vocational Qualifications (SVQs). There are four levels of NVQ, with Level 1 the most basic. Each level is made up of a number of units, covering the various beauty techniques as well as other aspects of the work. There is a lot more about NVQs and SVQs, as well as other qualifications, in Chapter 7 – 'Training day'.

# access to

## BEAUTY THERAPY

Look at the career paths below and decide which one is right for you

### HIGH STREET SALON

COLLEGE LEAVER
ASSISTANT BEAUTY THERAPIST
BEAUTY THERAPIST
SENIOR BEAUTY THERAPIST
ASSISTANT SALON MANAGER
SALON MANAGER OR SALON OWNER
GROUP SALON MANAGER

### SALES CONSULTANT

COLLEGE LEAVER
COUNTER SALES ADVISER
COMPANY SALES REPRESENTATIVE/ PRODUCT TRAINER
COMPANY SALES MANAGER/ PRODUCT TRAINER
REGIONAL SALES MANAGER/ PRODUCT TRAINER
NATIONAL SALES MANAGER

### SPA/HEALTH FARM

COLLEGE LEAVER
JUNIOR SPA THERAPIST
SPA THERAPIST
SENIOR SPA THERAPIST
ASSISTANT SPA MANAGER
SPA MANAGER

### TEACHING

COLLEGE LEAVER
BEAUTY/SPA THERAPIST FOR APPROX 3-5 YEARS
PART-TIME COURSE TO QUALIFY IN FAETC* INCL ASSESSOR AWARDS WHILST GAINING EXPERIENCE TEACHING OR;
PART-TIME COURSE FOR CERTIFICATE IN EDUCATION INCL ASSESSOR AWARDS WHILST GAINING EXPERIENCE TEACHING
LECTURER/ASSESSOR - FE, PRIVATE OR WORK-BASED
INTERNAL VERIFIER/EXAMINER/ EXTERNAL VERIFIER

Or you may instead choose to follow a career in Make-up or Nail Technology if you choose these options within your NVQ

## BEAUTY CONSULTANT

This is a person employed on a cosmetics counter in a department store or large pharmacy to advise clients on skincare, make-up and perfume products. You are also expected to analyse clients' skin, carry out makeovers and give skincare and make-up lessons. To do this job, **not only does your appearance have to be perfect**, but you also need to have a **way with words**. The other aspect of the job is the retailing and promotion. A beauty consultant needs a keen eye for detail and the ability to arrange products attractively. There is also an element of paperwork, for example customer records and administration.

*To do this job, not only does your appearance have to be perfect, but you also need to have a way with words.*

### TRAINING

Some cosmetic companies offer their own training, which usually amounts to a week-long induction course. This will train you only in the company's own brands and will not usually be a nationally recognised qualification. It's advisable, therefore, to already have the basic grounding of a qualification, such as an NVQ in Beauty Consultancy. Awarding bodies such as the Vocational Training and Charitable Trust (VTCT), City & Guilds and the International Therapy Examinational Council (ITEC) offer suitable courses.

### PAY AND HOURS

Hours are in line with usual shop opening hours, and you will be expected to work at weekends. Salaries will rise according to experience, and many product houses offer incentives such as staff discounts and commission on sales.

## THE GOOD

Seeing customers walk out holding their head up high after you've given them a makeover or sold them some fantastic products can be a thrill. It is especially satisfying to see clients return to you time after time because they know that you can give sound advice and recognise their type of skin and individual needs.

## THE BAD

Being on your feet all day! Occasionally you may have a very demanding client, and having to ensure that your appearance remains immaculate all day, no matter how tired or busy you are, can be wearing, too. You must appear unflappable, capable and efficient with a ready smile and a polite manner, whatever!

## ADVICE FOR STUDENTS

Get a Saturday job behind the counter in a department store or large pharmacy so that you get a feel of the job and what it entails.

## SALON BEAUTY SPECIALIST/THERAPIST

Becoming a beauty specialist  (otherwise known as a

Training offered by a product company will not usually result in an NVQ, and therefore will not lead to a career in beauty therapy. So be sure that you know what your future aims are.

beautician or beauty specialist) is generally the first step towards being a beauty therapist and can be achieved in one year on a full-time basis, with the award of an NVQ Level 2 or equivalent. Some learners only want to achieve this level, deciding to concentrate on skincare, nail treatments, make-up, eye treatments and wax depilation rather than the additional skills offered at NVQ Level 3. Beauty therapists, who are trained to do treatments for all the body, must be qualified to NVQ Level 3 or equivalent.

A salon therapist will be expected to carry out a variety of treatments throughout the day. It is vital that booking times are kept to so that clients are not kept waiting in reception. Salons can be hectic, so you need a **calm, efficient manner** to deal with the high volume of clients you will deal with in just one day. In an eight-hour day you could carry out treatments on more than 20 clients!

**TRAINING**
There is a wide range of options, but typically a one- to two-year course full time at college will result in an NVQ Level 3. Other options are combined college and workplace training such as the Foundation and Advanced Apprenticeship schemes (see Chapter 7) or shorter courses at private colleges.

Once qualified at NVQ Level 3 as a beauty therapist, you could decide to:

● specialise in one of the treatments such as electrolysis or body work

- train to qualify in other areas of beauty and complementary therapies
- progress to Level 4 for a career in Beauty Management.

There is more about these job areas below.

**PAY AND HOURS**
Pay may be low to start with, but for experienced therapists who bring in a lot of money for the business the potential to earn a substantial wage is there, particularly if you are paid commission on top. See Chapter 4 for more about incomes.

*You're never bored in a busy salon because of the wide range of treatments you cover in one day.*

Therapists normally work a five-day week but some salons operate on six and seven days (yes, some even open on Sundays now!). If your salon is like this you will be expected to work a rota system whereby every member of staff takes a turn to work the unsociable hours, including late opening in the evenings. You will still be entitled to a fixed day off per week though, and your hours should not exceed employment guidelines.

**THE GOOD**
You're never bored in a busy salon because of the wide range of treatments you cover in one day. Each client and each treatment are always different. You also get to work with and meet many different people.

## THE BAD

At times you may be so busy, with achy legs and feet, with no time for even so much as a cup of tea, that you feel anything but calm. Imagine it – a client has turned up late and made you get behind with your other clients; the phone is ringing; the receptionist is at lunch; and behind your smile and calm exterior you could happily scream! Remember, though, the good does outweigh the bad!

## ADVICE FOR STUDENTS

After college, gain employment and experience in a salon that employs quite a few other staff, so that you learn from them. Try to stay in your first job for at least a year, as anything less doesn't look great on your CV. A year in one place will teach you a great deal about the industry. Accept any offer of short courses and workshops from your employer in order to update and extend your skills.

## NAIL TECHNICIAN

This job involves applying artificial nails to the surface of the natural nail by building up and sculpting. The chemical components used are powder and liquid but harden very quickly when exposed to the air, forming a very tough extension over the natural nail. Skills needed are **speed, accuracy** and **attention to detail**. It's not essential to be artistic, but it certainly helps, especially for nail art, which is the creation of funky up-to-the-minute looks with the use of paint, glitter and nail jewellery. However, more important is good training. Clients wanting nail extensions are those who bite their nails, have slow-growing nails with a tendency to break easily or who just like the look of them.

**TRAINING**

NVQ Levels 2 and 3 now offer training for nail technicians, covering the essential knowledge and practical assessments needed to gain access to the industry. Awarding bodies are listed in Chapter 9 along with details of their websites, where all courses can be viewed.

**PAY AND HOURS**

A newly qualified nail technician can expect the **National Minimum Wage** particularly if working in a salon or nail bar. Brilliant money is out there for top technicians, who are in demand for education, session work, magazine and photographic work. A highly experienced self-employed nail technician can earn in excess of £25,000, particularly if she is in demand for media work or is the owner of a nail bar.

Hours will tend to be fairly set if working in a salon, but self-employed work can be unsociable with long hours.

**THE GOOD**

There is the pleasure of seeing clients leave the salon with renewed confidence as they look down at their beautiful nails. If you are really successful, the job could take you all over the world, with super-model or celebrity clients. There is also the opportunity to pass on your expertise by training new nail technicians.

**THE BAD**

Sitting for long periods of time leant over a nail station can wreak havoc on your back and neck. Also the smells of the nail products can be very strong and overpowering. Good posture and ventilation are crucial.

**ADVICE FOR STUDENTS**

After training, shadow an experienced Nail Technician for a

couple of months, even if you don't get paid! This grounding will teach you so much more about the clients, high standards, speed and accuracy needed to get on in the business. Enter competitions if you can (see Chapter 9 – 'Resources'). If you win or get placed, this will give you free publicity for your skills and put your name and face on the industry map.

## MOBILE BEAUTY THERAPIST

Once you have trained and gained some salon experience, you may decide to branch out on your own. Mobile treatments require a lot of organisation, but are worth doing if you need to work around family commitments. If you are also wary of paying rent, then this is the way to go as long as you don't mind carrying around equipment from house to house. An important fact to remember is that you could end up covering unnecessary miles if you don't work out your routes and **organise yourself** to work within a certain area for a particular day or period of time. The range of clients is wide, but quite a large proportion of business can come from care homes and hospitals, mothers at home with small children and the disabled and elderly. So ensure that you target this large client group with your advertising methods. Alternatively you could set up a home practice if you prefer a base to work from.

### TRAINING

The usual recognised Beauty Therapy training – a minimum of NVQ/SVQ Level 2 – is needed.

### PAY AND HOURS

The pay really depends on you. If you are very businesslike with your scheduling, travel arrangements and appointment bookings, you can successfully earn a very good salary.

Remember, though, the best advertising is word of mouth, so keep those clients happy!

The hours, too, can vary – remember that mobile therapists can do a lot of their work in the evenings when people have finished work and want a relaxing evening at home having a massage. The popular thing nowadays is pamper parties where a hostess arranges for a few friends to come around and have treatments by a beauty therapist.

### THE GOOD
The overheads are low – just the running of your vehicle (plus electricity if home-based), as well as product costs. You are also in control of your working hours and what you do with them.

### THE BAD
It can be lonely working on your own, especially when you are faced with a problem or important decision and there's no one with you to advise you. It can also involve lots of driving around and carrying heavy equipment in all weathers. There is also the less pleasant aspect of working at home after normal working hours because you will need to do your bookkeeping and accounts, stock checking and ordering, equipment cleaning and maintenance and laundry.

### ADVICE FOR STUDENTS
Don't expect to be able to work alone straight from college, you need the experience of salon work. If you eventually decide to go mobile, then check out the area – is it needed? If you know someone in a different area that does mobile treatments, ask for their advice. Finally, speak to a small-business adviser and get as much information about running your own business

as you can. Have a separate telephone number apart from your home one, otherwise you will find yourself called on at all hours – a mobile for business is the best solution.

Be strict about your treatment time. Tell clients how long you expect the treatment to take and that you will need to leave by a certain time. Clients answering calls and seeing to the family will eat into your time and end up costing you money and making you late for your next appointment. Choose your products and equipment carefully – the equipment must be hard-wearing and the products (such as wax) where possible should be water-based to facilitate cleaning if spilt.

## WORKING ON CRUISE LINERS

Jobs in this field are available for beauty therapists, massage therapists and nail technicians. You will be working in a top-class establishment, albeit on the waves. You will be expected to get on with everyone, both the 1,000–3,000 passengers and the 500–1,500 crew members. So the **ability to work in a team** is essential. Each contract is for approximately eight months, and during this time you will share an extremely small cabin with another spa team member. You are required to be **physically and emotionally healthy**. You must have a medical before joining ship.

**DID YOU KNOW?**

There are approximately 8,000 beauty salons in the UK.

### TRAINING

Beauty therapists must be qualified to Level 3 standard with one of the recognised awarding bodies. Facial and body massage, including electrical face and body treatments, is essential.

Massage therapists must be qualified in Swedish massage with a recognised qualification. Additional qualifications in therapies such as shiatsu, reflexology, reiki, sports massage and aromatherapy are a great advantage.

Nail technicians must be qualified with good industrial experience in all nail-enhancement systems (for example gel and acrylic). They also need to be qualified in Manicure and Pedicure. An NVQ Level 2 and 3 or recognised nail technician course is expected.

### PAY AND HOURS
Hours can be long, and you will be expected to do shift work so that flexible working patterns can be arranged to cover evening work. The pay depends on your position on board and your experience. However, most of your earnings will come from commission. Tips from passengers can seriously increase your earnings.

### THE GOOD
Career prospects and opportunities for promotion within the company are good. There will be the chance to see places around the world as you will get some time off at ports of call.

### THE BAD
Sharing what is little more than a cupboard as a bedroom can be taxing. On board ship you are never off-duty. The fast-paced life can be hectic and stressful, as is being away from home for such a long period of time. Homesickness and seasickness are both very possible!

### ADVICE FOR STUDENTS
If this is a longer-term goal, you should first complete your

beauty-therapy training and go into industry for a couple of years in order to develop a mature outlook and treatment experience. During this time, try to expand your skills with further training in order to give you a head start above other job candidates. Start applying to cruise-liner companies six months before you want to start so that you have time to attend interviews and have medicals. Interviews are ongoing and UK-wide.

## AIRLINE THERAPIST

This is physically demanding work, as you will be on your feet constantly during flights. You must be friendly, approachable and polite at all times. You must be technically excellent because the treatments are carried out on First Class passengers who expect the best. Even after a long-haul flight **your grooming must be immaculate**. You will fly mainly from Heathrow. A company medical and excellent health is essential as is a preliminary training course. You must be 19–33 years of age, 5' 2" minimum in height, fluent in English and a holder of a European Union passport, as well as having salon experience of at least one year.

### TRAINING

NVQ/SVQ Level 3 or equivalent standard from an awarding body is expected.

### PAY AND HOURS

Airlines offer a good salary package, which includes flight allowances and commission payments. Holiday is 28 days per year. After complying with certain criteria, you will also be offered concessionary travel, private medical insurance and pension schemes.

### THE GOOD
You'll have global travel opportunities and the chance to meet friends and interesting people.

### THE BAD
There will be long tiring flights and some demanding passengers, and you will have to take your turn to work bank holidays, including Christmas. Remember the unsociable hours can disrupt your social life.

### ADVICE FOR STUDENTS
Go into industry, gain experience and then apply to an airline through its website. They are unable to reply personally if you have been unsuccessful, but don't be put off – you may be more successful next time. Just keep trying!

## SALON OWNER
For this profile, we will assume that you are a qualified beauty therapist, simply because you would not have the skills, understanding and background knowledge to run your own beauty salon and a team of staff – unless you employed a beauty therapist as the day-to-day manager.

Being your own boss is not necessarily the best option; it can mentally and physically exhausting and can try your patience at the best of times.

Competition between salons can be fierce, but if yours is well run, with quality treatments being carried out, you can succeed. As owner, you would be expected to carry out treatments, organise staff rotas, carry out payroll paperwork and wages, complete monthly and end-of-year accounts, order stock, stocktake, interview and employ new staff, arrange PR and advertising and much more. Your day would start before the staff arrive and finish after they have gone home. Being your own boss is not necessarily the best option; it can be mentally and physically exhausting and can try your patience at the best of times.

**TRAINING**
Level 3 Beauty Therapy or equivalent is the basic, while a management qualification is a definite advantage.

**PAY AND HOURS**
This can vary enormously, depending on how busy the salon is, where the business is situated, how many staff you need to pay and so on. It is best to set yourself a small salary, and at the year end see what profit has been made, what equipment needs to be replaced, which staff need pay rises and what decoration and alterations need doing before finally deciding whether to increase your salary.

**THE GOOD**
You will hopefully get a great sense of satisfaction from what you have achieved, especially if your business is thriving and you have a sense of pride in what you do.

**THE BAD**
Long hours, sorting out staff problems or disagreements and managing paperwork and administration are just a few of the headaches. Another is the worry when the business hits a slow period of the year and bookings fall.

## ADVICE FOR STUDENTS

Don't even think about setting up your own business until you have had a few jobs and experienced the good and not so good ways that salons are run. Take it all in, hone your skills and learn as much as you can about the non-treatment side of beauty therapy. Undertake a management course whilst working in a salon.

## ELECTROLYSIST

This job involves treating unwanted hair growth by inserting a fine sterile needle into the hair follicle and passing a mild, controlled electrical current through it to the root of the hair. This cauterises the hair-production area, which enables the hair to be lifted out by forceps (electrolysis tweezers). This is a gradual weakening process that destroys the hair over a number of treatments.

You must have **excellent interpersonal skills** as the treatment can be very intimate, involving close work and knowledge of the client's medical history. Clients are often very self-conscious of their hair growth and need to be put at ease from the start. Comprehensive knowledge of the skin and hair and of health and safety are essential, as is **good eyesight** and **steady hands**.

### TRAINING

You can follow the NVQ Level 3 general route; choose the Epilation unit as an additional option if taking an alternative Level 3 route (for example Spa or Nail Services) or take another appropriate examination course. Awarding bodies such as VTCT, City & Guilds, Edexcel and ITEC offer suitable courses. Membership of the British Association of Electrolysists (see Chapter 9 for contact details) is subject to an additional examination as it expects standards to be very high.

## PAY AND HOURS
Pay is in line with salon wages for the level of experience unless you are self-employed. Working as an electrolysist on a mobile basis is not particularly financially viable as many of the sessions are short, as little as ten minutes at a time. It is far better to work from a base such as home or as a chair-renter. Hours are quite standard unless self-employed, in which case you will be expected to carry out some evening work.

## THE GOOD
The emotional boost a client gets from seeing her unwanted hair disappearing from her face is enormous. It gives the therapist a huge boost, too, to see how she has helped a client who may have been lacking in self-esteem and social confidence.

It gives the therapist a huge boost to see how she has helped a client who may have been lacking in self-esteem and social confidence.

## THE BAD
Such close work involving accuracy and concentration can affect the eyes over a period of time. This may just be eyestrain or occasional headaches. If good posture is not maintained, back and neck problems can occur.

## ADVICE FOR STUDENTS

Develop your skills in the workplace first, and then apply for membership to the Institute. The British Association of Electrolysists gives out names of its members to potential clients looking for practitioners in their area, keeps you informed of new developments and holds seminars for professional development.

## CAMOUFLAGE MAKE-UP SPECIALIST

In this job, you will cover birthmarks, scars, accident injuries and burns using corrective make-up techniques and specialist make-up. The job could be freelance, going where the work takes you. A lot of the work could be hospital-based in special units.

### TRAINING

This subject is a unit within Level 3 Beauty Therapy courses. This will provide you with the necessary background knowledge of the skin and anatomy as well as the basics of make-up before you move into more specialised and sensitive topics.

### PAY AND HOURS

If freelance, pay and hours could vary greatly as you will be doing your own costings. If employed, however, they will follow the requirements of the NMW as a minimum.

### THE GOOD

You will get enormous job satisfaction from seeing people cosmetically improved where once they had disfiguring marks that caused them great distress and embarrassment.

**THE BAD**

Some disfigurements can be distressful to the onlooker. You need to remember that it's just visual and your job is to improve the appearance of it for the client.

**ADVICE FOR STUDENTS**

Contact the National Health Service (NHS) and private hospitals for information about remedial camouflage. They will be able to advise you as to the best way to go. Usually you can't go wrong if you shadow an experienced person. This will give you both experience and contacts.

## SALES REPRESENTATIVE

A sales representative is employed by a product, equipment or cosmetic company to sell its goods to salons and spas nationally or regionally. The job involves a lot of travelling around, meeting prospective suppliers and answering their queries. You must be completely knowledgeable about the product that you are promoting and sincerely believe in it yourself. Your attitude must be **professional, efficient** and **organised**. There will also be an element of paperwork, such as appointment scheduling, record-keeping and sales data.

**TRAINING**

A beauty therapy or consultancy background is ideal so that you have the essential knowledge of the industry and salon/spa requirements for business success. Once you have experience as a therapist or consultant, knowledge in various brands will also stand you in good stead. For example, if you undertook extra training in a range of skincare brands you would be at an advantage if a job were advertised for the particular brand you had trained in.

### PAY AND HOURS

These can vary, but sales representatives are usually offered a yearly salary with commission on sales. A company car and other benefits such as discounts and healthcare can also be offered.

### THE GOOD

Being independent is a plus. You get to make your own appointments, research your area and follow up contacts which, when good, can lead to a big sale or a company account on the books.

### THE BAD

On a bad day, you could be travelling around all day without anyone being interested in taking on the product.

### ADVICE FOR STUDENTS

Get experience as a beauty consultant or beauty/spa therapist and, whilst working, undertake continuous development in new/existing treatments and products so that you are ready for when the particular company you are interested in is recruiting.

## DID YOU KNOW?

British Beauty Therapy is recognised as the best in the world.

### SPORTS MASSAGE THERAPIST

The job involves massage and manipulation of the muscles and joints. The massage itself is much deeper and more intense than a Swedish massage and **you need a strong physique and hands**, as the work is very physically demanding. Sports massage is a special form of massage and is typically used before, during and after athletic events. The purpose of the massage is to prepare the athlete for peak performance, to drain away fatigue, to relieve swelling, to reduce muscle tension, to promote flexibility and to prevent injuries. Sports massage can help prevent those niggling injuries that so often get in the way of performance and achievement, whether a person is an athlete or a once-a-week jogger.

**TRAINING**
You will need to achieve a qualification in Anatomy, Physiology and Body Massage before advancing to a Sports Massage qualification from a recognised awarding body.

**PAY AND HOURS**
Sports massage is usually offered in health clubs and fitness centres or as a freelance service and occasionally in hospitals. If you're lucky, you can be assigned to work for a sports team as their sports massage therapist. If you have a good reputation, then you can expect to charge a good hourly rate that takes into account your expertise. There may be a lot of weekend work, especially if you are part of a sports team.

**THE GOOD**
Job satisfaction may come from alleviating a person's pain and discomfort or from treating muscles to keep them fit and healthy.

**THE BAD**
This is a very strenuous job that can cause aches and pains in you if you don't maintain correct posture. Freelancing also involves a lot of driving around to clients, sometimes at very unsociable hours. You go where and when you are needed.

### ADVICE FOR STUDENTS

Whilst training, volunteer your services to a local team at the weekend so that you can practise your sports massage skills. If they already have a qualified person, then ask if you can shadow them. You will pick up lots of good techniques and advice.  Alternatively ask a local health club, fitness centre or physiotherapy department in a hospital if you can do work experience for them.

## MAKE-UP ARTIST

You may intend to specialise in theatrical, media or television and film make-up, but if you have a wealth of experience behind you, you could become an all-rounder. There are general differences between the areas, but a lot of the skills tend to overlap at times.

Theatrical make-up involves applying period and costume make-up for plays and productions and very often very elaborate fantasy make-up. Just think of the musical *Cats!* Media involves making up actors, celebrities, models and presenters, along with carrying out high-fashion make-up for magazine work, photographic shoots and platform/runway shows. Television and film make-up involves much of the above plus designing and making prosthetics. Prosthetics are false facial and body features that change the appearance of an actor.

A large part of make-up artistry involves hair, as wigs, hairpieces, beards and moustaches are also used, so a hairdressing qualification would give you a distinct advantage. Many employers in this area of the industry will not employ you without one. You will certainly also need a **good sense of colour**, balance and design. **Creativity is**

*You will certainly also need a good sense of colour, balance and design. Creativity is essential, as is tact and patience, as you will be working within a demanding industry.*

**essential**, as is **tact** and **patience**, as you will be working within a demanding industry. You must be able to work under pressure and have good communication skills.

**TRAINING**
The starting point is qualifications in Beauty and Hairdressing, especially as NVQ Beauty now offers the make-up route. You would then need to take a course in TV and film make-up or be an apprentice to a freelance make-up artist so that you can learn the trade first hand.

**PAY AND HOURS**
Hours can vary greatly. You need to take the work as it comes because if you freelance you may have long periods without assignments. The pay can be excellent particularly if you're in demand. You will be working for a daily fee, which usually starts from about £250.

**THE GOOD**
There's the possibility of extensive travel to exotic places, meeting famous people, seeing your work on the big screen, and seeing your name credited in magazines, shows and television. Working on such a wide variety of projects and assignments makes it hard to get bored.

**THE BAD**
The job can involve a lot of standing around and waiting, especially in the TV and film industry. You'll be under pressure to work to strict timescales and you will need to fit in around other people. A lot of the people that you make up are very demanding and can test your patience.

**ADVICE FOR STUDENTS**
GCSEs in subjects such as Art, History and Human Anatomy would be very helpful. Be prepared to work unpaid in amateur dramatics and local theatre companies to gain experience and build up a portfolio to show prospective employees.

**DID YOU KNOW?**

Jesse Wallace, who plays Kat Slater in 'EastEnders', trained as a make-up artist before becoming an actor.

**HOLISTIC THERAPIST**
In this job, you might specialise in Indian head massage, aromatherapy or reflexology, or even be qualified to offer all.

Aromatherapy uses blends of essential oils that have been extracted from flowers, trees, spices, fruit or herbs. The oils have healing and relaxing properties and can be applied by massage, baths, compresses and inhalations. Aromatherapy is also used in hospitals to boost ill patients.

Indian head massage is based on traditional Indian techniques that use a variety of massage movements. It is a unique and versatile treatment involving massage of the scalp, neck and shoulders to induce relaxation and a feeling of well-being.

Reflexology uses specialised massage techniques on the soles of the feet. The soles represent a mirror image or map of the body, and by massaging parts of the feet you can unblock energy pathways and alleviate minor ailments in the body. It is best used as a preventative measure against more serious ailments.

## TRAINING

There are no specific entry requirements to train as a holistic therapist. However, some courses expect you to have a basic massage qualification first. You will also be expected to learn about the anatomy and physiology of the body. This may be a separate course that runs alongside the practical part, or it may be built into the qualification, depending on the award that you are studying for. There are many courses available, both private and state-run, but make sure that if you study privately the course is a recognised and endorsed qualification or you will not be able to obtain insurance.

## PAY AND HOURS

If you are mobile, then the hours you work are your choice, but because of the popularity of holistic treatments you could be in great demand. The cost of the treatment to the client can range from £20 to £40. The nature of holistic therapies demands that the treatment be carried out in a calm and stress-free manner and environment, so rushing from one client to the next is not going to work. In a salon or spa you can expect to earn the minimum wage upwards, depending on your experience and position.

## THE GOOD

The satisfaction comes from seeing how you can turn a wound-up, stressed-out client into a relaxed, chilled-out person before they leave. It is a modern-day fact that high levels of stress are causing illness and even shortening our lives, so feeling that you have played a part in cutting down that stress can give you an enormous sense of satisfaction.

**THE BAD**
Holistic therapy is a very giving treatment and can be very emotionally draining, especially if you are carrying out six holistic treatments in one day.

**ADVICE FOR STUDENTS**
Get experience in the industry first – as a masseur or beauty therapist – to gain experience with clients. Holistic therapists need a very mature attitude and a high level of life experience in order to be in a position to offer these type of treatments successfully and for a client to feel at ease with them.

*The satisfaction comes from seeing how you can turn a wound-up, stressed-out client into a relaxed, chilled-out person before they leave.*

**WRITER**
This could take the form of a staff writer on a health and beauty magazine, a freelance journalist specialising in beauty or an author of educational books and materials for a publisher. You must be prepared to work to tight deadlines. It can be very interesting work because you get the low-down on all the new products, techniques and training.

You need a **good knowledge of the English language** and good word-processing and keyboard skills. Be prepared to carry out extensive research to ensure that you write accurate and up-to-date material. You need to have a **determined personality** in order to be able to take the rejection of material returned or refused. Don't give up!

## TRAINING
A good background in Beauty Therapy is essential, so you will probably need to qualify in NVQ/SVQ Beauty Level 2 minimum. A course in writing and journalism is advisable, as is a GCSE in English.

## PAY AND HOURS
This varies enormously depending on whether you are writing a book or just a column in a magazine. If you write books and are paid on a royalty basis, the industry average is 10 per cent of net receipt (sales), or you could be paid a one-off fee for the book instead. For information on magazine and periodical rates, *The Writer's Handbook* edited by Barry Turner is a good guide as it also lists all the magazines and newspapers in the UK and Europe. Hours can be long if you are working to a deadline.

## THE GOOD
You may like working under your own steam and being able to do some writing jobs around your family commitments. Seeing your writing actually in print gives you a great sense of satisfaction.

## THE BAD
There's the tight, sore muscles in the neck and shoulders from being sat at a computer for so many hours, and

sometimes you have to burn the midnight oil to get work finished. Additional hazards are the possible repetitive strain injury from using the keyboard and eyestrain from staring at a computer screen for long periods of time.

### ADVICE FOR STUDENTS
Visit publishers' and magazine houses' websites to check out their jobs and submission advice. Check out *The Writer's Handbook* for companies that accept samples of your writing. Alternatively, ask to do work experience on a magazine so that you get some useful contacts as well as seeing how the system works. For training in magazine journalism, visit the website of the Periodicals Training Council at www.ppa.co.uk/ptc.

## DID YOU KNOW?

Currently there are about 500 approved training providers for Hair and Beauty offering Beauty qualifications in the UK alone.

### LECTURER/TRAINER
You can work as a company/product trainer or get a part-time or full-time job in a private or further education (FE) college. The groups of students that you teach can vary in size from one to 18, but the important thing is that you must have the ability to impart information in a clear, accurate and interesting way. Your methods must be **well planned** and **organised**. You also need a firm but fair hand in order to maintain a professional level of conduct in teaching salons where there are actual paying clients.

### TRAINING
You will have completed your basic training and achieved NVQ/SVQ Level 3 in Beauty Therapy. After gaining a few

years' experience you then need to attend a part-time course at college to gain the Further and Adult Education Teachers Certificate (FAETC), which gives you the basic grounding in how to teach students, plan your lessons and organise your class. You may then decide to progress to a teaching degree such as a Post Graduate Certificate in Education (PGCE) or a Certificate in Education (Cert Ed). You will be expected to carry out teaching practice during your training and will be assessed on your competence in teaching students.  When training for a teaching qualification, you will also be expected to gain an assessor award, without which you will not be able to assess students.

**PAY AND HOURS**
A full-time salary in an FE college rises with experience – the range is from approximately £10,000 to £30,000. Private colleges will have their own salary scale, and if you are a part-time lecturer you will be paid hourly.

**THE GOOD**
Getting groups of students through their qualification can give you a real kick – seeing how they have developed from day one until they graduate, and feeling that you had a lot to do with their achievements.

**THE BAD**
There's lots of preparation, marking and paperwork, much of which you will have to take home to complete. Although the holidays may seem long, it is extremely rare for you not to have to take work home with you during these breaks. Then there's dealing with the odd stroppy learner who doesn't think that 'good practice' and occupational standards apply to them!

**ADVICE FOR STUDENTS**

You will need to gain a few years experience in the industry before you even think about teaching. Approach a few educational establishments to sound out their recruitment methods – as always, a bit of shadowing does no harm for picking up tips and contacts.

## MAKING YOUR MIND UP

You should now have a good idea of the wealth of opportunities that exist in the beauty industry. Perhaps you've already decided which direction you would like to go in – you might always have known! – but if you're still unsure, you may find it useful to visit two government careers websites – www.connexions.gov.uk/occupations and www.educationuk.org. Both sites are excellent sources of careers advice for the student wishing to pursue a career in the beauty field.

*Now you've got another choice to make – where are you going to get that all-important training?*

2

# How to get in and on in the beauty industry

By now you should have more of an idea whether a career in Beauty is for you. There is the right job and training for everyone interested in the beauty industry. The most difficult choice is where and how to train and deciding on which career path to take. In this chapter, you'll find some more about how to track down the right course for you. On page 36, there's an easy-to-follow flow chart showing the whole process of interviewing and enrolling for a course. There's also more about training in Chapter 7.

## CHOOSING A GOOD TRAINING CENTRE

With a wide range of Beauty Therapy courses available and many different training centres to choose from, where do you start? When looking at a college prospectus or phoning for information to a training centre, this is what the Hairdressing and Beauty Industry Authority (HABIA) advises prospective students to investigate:

- the number of students on the course and the staff/student ratio
- the length of the course and whether it's full or part time
- whether it's free and whether you would be eligible for a grant
- whether you qualify for tax relief on the training fee or a career development loan, if you are paying
- whether the course leads to an NVQ/SVQ in Hairdressing or Beauty Therapy or any other approved qualification in the National Qualification Framework
- what level the course will reach
- how many students were on the course last year, how many achieved the required level and how many of them got jobs
- whether you can complete the course unit by unit, returning at a convenient time to complete any outstanding units
- what will be expected of you in terms of daily/weekly/monthly assessments and exams
- how much equipment is provided and how much additional equipment will cost
- whether you can have a look around the college or training centre and meet for a chat with the trainers and current students
- the enrolment procedure – can you enrol at any time or are there set dates?
- whether you will be given a placement in a local salon to develop your skills, or be expected to find one yourself
- what options for training routes are available
- whether the centre has a quality award from an external organisation, such as a Chartermark or National Training Award.

You'll need to weigh up the advantages and disadvantages of what's available and decide on the training option that suits your circumstances best. Remember, your college entrance interview is a chance for you to find out more about the course just as much as it is a chance for them to find out about you! Be prepared to ask questions, such as whether there are grants available or whether there's childcare. This type of information may well help you in your decision-making. Below, we'll take look at some of the issues listed above in a bit more detail.

## PART TIME OR FULL TIME?

Being a full-time student is not the only way to learn. If you're working, unemployed or have family commitments, you can still study and get qualifications. Part-time and home study requires a lot of self-discipline, though, especially when you need to fit it around the demands of your home and work life. But if you've got the determination, you can do it.

Choosing whether to study part or full time is crucial because rules about whether you pay and how much you pay for a course depend on this. It may also affect the kind of support you get for living expenses. Think things through carefully.

Being a full-time student is not the only way to learn. If you're working, unemployed or have family commitments, you can still study and get qualifications.

# ENTRY TO COLLEGE

### TELEPHONE OR CALL IN FOR A PROSPECTUS

### CHOOSE A COURSE

### COMPLETE THE APPLICATION FORM

## ATTEND A COURSE INTERVIEW AND COLLEGE VISIT

- Immaculate appearance and positive attitude
- Take Record of Achievement to be looked through and or references if adult learner
- Questions prepared about the course etc
- Will be given information on course fees and financial help

## LETTER OF ACCEPTANCE

Should detail:
- date of enrolment
- place and time of enrolment
- what to bring

## ENROLMENT

- Enrolment paperwork completed
- Course start date and times given
- Some colleges arrange facility for kit and uniform purchase at this
- May be given recommended book reading list

### START OF TERM

Basically, for state-run education you need to remember that

- if you are under 19 and studying full time you won't usually have to pay any course fees
- if you're 19 or over but claiming state benefits (or on a pension) you may be exempt from course fees or be able to pay at a reduced rate
- if you're working and you want to take a course that will help you in your current job, your employer may be willing to help out
- if you're 16 or 17 and working you may have the right to time off for study
- the government offers training programmes like Apprenticeships and National Traineeships that give young people the chance to get qualifications while earning a wage or training allowance. Ask at your local Careers Centre or go to www.jobcentreplus.gov.uk.

The situation with regard to support and fees payment for part-time day or evening courses is more complicated:

- It's worth approaching the Student Awards Department of your Local Education Authority (LEA), who may be able to offer financial support for part-time students.
- If you're unemployed and claiming benefit you may still be able to study part time during the day up to a certain number of hours without it affecting your claim, under the New Deal Programme. Check with your Jobcentre or Benefits Office.
- You may be able to get a Jobseeker's Allowance if you are studying part time.
- If you are working for an employer, there are training allowances available for employees.

Once again, don't be shy about going to your local Careers Centre to find out more. Look at www.jobcentreplus.gov.uk.

## WHAT WILL I NEED TO PAY FOR?

When choosing a course you need to look carefully at what exactly you will have to pay for – not only in terms of the course itself but also the 'incidentals', such as travelling expenses and childcare. Expenses could include:

- registration fees
- specialist equipment (e.g. essential tools for beauty therapy)
- professional clothing (uniforms and shoes)
- general study materials, including photocopying, printing, computer discs and so on
- daily or weekly transport to college sites
- childcare (see the box on page 40)
- travel to work placements, day visits or study tours
- general living expenses (accommodation, food and so on)
- fees for learning programmes (courses) and exam fees.

Although it is often difficult to meet all the costs of studying, it can be useful to find out any likely costs before you start a course. Some learning programmes or courses will be more expensive than others. Remember, you are entitled to ask for information about the costs of your particular course or programme, and colleges should provide written information and advice on fees, costs and student finance.

The costs can seem daunting, but don't panic! You should be able to get financial help with many of these things.

## FINANCIAL HELP

Many part-time courses have reduced or concessionary fees. To be eligible, you must be in receipt of a means-tested benefit or be the unwaged dependant of someone who is receiving a benefit. To apply for fee reduction, you must enrol in person (or send photocopied details), so you can prove that you are genuinely entitled to reduced fees.

### SPREADING THE COST

It may also possible to pay in instalments for programmes costing more than £200 that are more than one term in length. A first payment of 50 per cent of fees payable on enrolment and two subsequent instalments on the first day of the following two months can be arranged.

### TRAVEL

Colleges provide travel passes (bus or rail) for full-time students under the age of 19 years at the start of their course. You pay the first £30 of travel costs to and from college per term and the college pays the rest, up to a maximum of £210. Students whose parents receive a means-tested state benefit get the travel pass free of charge.

### EXAMINATION FEES

Students in receipt of a means-tested benefit or the unwaged dependant of someone in receipt of benefits can also get help with paying for examination fees. Ask your college guidance centre for details.

### LOAN ADVICE

The college guidance centre can also help you with a Career Development Loan. This may sound a bit scary, but it could be a sensible option – think of it as investing in your future.

Career Development Loans are a way of borrowing money to finance learning and have a special low interest rate. You can borrow anything from £300 to £8,000, which can be used to fund up to two years of learning plus up to one year's practical work experience where it forms part of the course. The Department for Education and Skills (DfES) pays the interest on your loan while you're learning and for up to one month afterwards. You then repay the loan to the bank over an agreed period at a fixed rate of interest. For more information on Career Development Loans, ring 0800 585 505 or visit www.lifelonglearning.co.uk/cdl.

---

**WHAT ABOUT CHILDCARE?**

There may be some childcare places available at some colleges, but there are usually never enough, so speak to student services staff who may be able to help with suggestions. On some New Deal programmes, there may be funds available for childcare. Some other courses or learning programmes may also include an allowance for childcare, or you may be able to get some help from college learning support, access or welfare funds.

---

In some colleges or universities, you may be eligible for a small amount of money from the Access Fund or from any college welfare fund, learner support fund or hardship fund, if they exist at your place of study.

## HELP AND GUIDANCE

You're probably thinking that there's a lot to take in here.

There is, and it could well make sense to get further advice. Initially, it's probably best to ask staff at student services in the college. Do this as early as possible – **when you apply**. Don't wait until you enrol. Other sources of information and advice include your local Citizens Advice Bureau, welfare rights advisers in your local authority and your local library. There's also an extensive list of resources in Chapter 9, which should provide you with many other leads.

## CONGRATULATIONS – YOU'VE BEEN ACCEPTED!

Beauty Therapy courses are vocational, which means that they are preparing you for the job that you will eventually do. So you need to remember that Industry Codes of Practice and conforming to regulations must start here. Your conduct, dress code and health and safety must be first rate. The job is providing a service to the public, and there is no room for sloppy service and can't-care-less attitudes.

You should look on a training centre for a vocational course as your employer. For example, don't be late for lessons and don't take sickies! Work as a team and respect your fellow students – this way you will be prepared for entry into a hard-working industry that thrives on its good reputation.

> **DID YOU KNOW?**
>
> Currently there are about 500 approved training providers offering beauty qualifications in the UK alone, both in further education colleges and in the private sector.

Now – imagine you've completed your course and you've graduated with flying colours. You've qualified, you're eager to get on with a real job in the beauty industry, you want to show the world what you're capable of. The next hurdle, then, is to find a job, and this is what we'll cover in the next chapter.

# Job hunting for the beauty graduate

You've spotted an advertisement for your dream job, so what do you do next? In this chapter, we'll look at an overview of the process of applying for jobs and the interview process. For more detailed advice and information, you could also take a look at *Winning Interviews for First-time Job Hunters* and *Winning CVs for First-time Job Hunters* (2nd edition), both by Kath Houston, published by Trotman.

When job hunting, you will need to be organised. If you need to update your details, type out a letter of introduction or gather your certificates together, do this in good time. Job applications have closing dates, and if your application arrives just one day late, you will not get your chance to shine. Your application will probably not even be looked at, even if you *really are* the perfect person for the job.

It is important that you make sure your CV and covering letter shines. Present yourself in your CV and covering letters as you will do in your professional life: immaculately and honestly.

Another possibility when job hunting is to use the services of a recruitment agency. See the box on page 44 and the list in

Chapter 9 for more on recruitment companies specialising in the health and beauty industry.

---

**RECRUITMENT COMPANIES**

Recruitment companies specialise in matching the right candidate to the right job. Preparing your CV, writing the covering letter and developing your interview techniques are three of the most important stages in progressing your career, and they can advise you on this as well as help you find a job.

You need to register your details and current CV. This is usually free, and there is no obligation to accept the job that they match you with if, for example, something better comes along. Recruitment specialists usually charge the company that they have managed to find an employee for rather than the employee themselves, although this can vary. They will want to interview you, too – and all the advice given below about interviews applies here as well.

---

## CVs, LETTERS AND APPLICATION FORMS

Application forms, CVs and covering letters are used in order to introduce yourself to the employer. Some jobs have hundreds of people applying for them so it's important that you stand out from the crowd. From the hundreds of job applications, just a few will be short-listed for an interview. Here are a few of the dos and don'ts when sending in an application for a job –

- Read the job advert very carefully – it's essential that you do exactly what the advert says. This may sound obvious, but it is surprising how many people ignore the instructions. For example, if an advert asks you to phone for further details in the first instance then do just that, don't send in your CV instead. All companies have their own format for recruitment, and if you get it wrong at first base what hope do you have of making a good impression?

- When putting together your CV, don't follow a model CV (for example, from a book or the Internet) slavishly. Make sure that you have added your own personal touch.

- One CV is not enough for a lifetime! Your education, work history and skills will develop over time, and it is essential that you update your CV yearly and that you also tailor it to each different job or purpose.

- In the beauty industry it is practical experience and good-quality college training that impress. Because salons and spas rely heavily on repeat bookings, they will be looking for candidates who don't have a history of moving about from job to job too regularly. Advertising the fact that you have worked in six different places in two years is not good!

If the company likes your cover letter, CV or application, they will select you for an interview. This is called short-listing.

## INTERVIEWS

The interview could be with one person or with a panel of interviewers. The latter can be very daunting but, however many interviewers there are, you need to stay calm and look professional. It's about acting confidently and showing yourself in the best possible light.

In an interview panel for a beauty job, you might expect to find the manager – who wants to make sure that you would fit in with the team, perhaps the head therapist – who wants to ensure that your occupational standards and approach to client care are second to none and, in larger businesses, someone from Human Resources, which is responsible for the recruitment process.

Put aside time before the interview to find out a bit about the company and the job you are going for. Practise some typical interview questions and answers with a friend, and have ready a few of your own questions, such as 'Who will I report to?' or 'When will I know whether I have been selected?'. Practise the journey to the interview, time it and then still leave early on the day – just in case!

Before you set out, make sure that you have everything you need with you to prove that you have the right qualifications and experience – for example certificates or diplomas or a record of achievement if you are a school-leaver or student. If you are doing trade tests, you will also need to have your equipment, tools and uniform (more on this below).

The most important things to remember for an interview are:

- smile and be friendly
- be yourself and never pretend to be someone you are not; it will be hard to live up to if you are selected
- maintain good posture when walking into the room and sitting down
- use positive body language with good eye contact
- sit only when invited to and don't slouch in the seat
- don't smoke (even beforehand – your clothes will smell) or chew gum.

Appearance is crucial in an interview for a job in the beauty industry. Remember that you will be almost a walking advert for the company's services or products. You need to:

- wear smart, clean, ironed clothes and polished shoes
- make sure you wear well-applied day make-up; it definitely should not be heavy
- make sure your nails are well manicured and fairly short; long or artificial nails when interviewing for a job as a Beauty Therapist will be a real turn-off for employers
- make sure your hair is neat, clean and free from split ends or roots growing out.

When answering questions, always have the evidence ready to back up your statements and claims. If, for example, the interviewer asks you whether you are good at working in a team, make sure you can back this up with an instance where you have shown this – whether in a job or at college or somewhere else.

If you get to the interview stage but are unsuccessful, make sure you ask for feedback as to why you were not selected. You can use their comments to improve when applying for your next position.

Here are a few good examples of strengths and weaknesses to identify in interview. Always be ready to give an example of where you have shown any strengths that you mention:

**STRENGTHS**
- good timekeeping
- ability to get on with people and work as a team
- professional attitude
- organisational skills.

**WEAKNESSES**
- a bit of a perfectionist, like everything to be in order
- spending too much money on clothes and beauty magazines.

These weakness could turn to your advantage and be looked on as strengths, because they show that you like things to be organised and just right; also that you keep up-to-date with beauty and fashion.

## TRADE TESTS

Because beauty therapy is a practical occupation, part of the interview process will include what is known as a 'trade test' or 'skills test'. This is when you will be asked to demonstrate a practical treatment on someone so that the company can view your practical skills and techniques. This is often done at a second interview after the company has first seen you, talked to you and felt that you could fit in as part of the team.

Immaculate appearance and hygiene are essential during a trade test.

Trade tests can be a very nerve-racking experience, but don't worry – interviewers will usually take nerves into consideration in their assessment of you. Some employers will let you know beforehand which treatments you will be expected to carry out on the day. This is a much fairer system as it allows you time to prepare, which in turn will help to calm your nerves.

Again, immaculate appearance and hygiene are essential during a trade test. You should wear a clean and ironed uniform, along with clean, sensible shoes. Your hair should be tied back neatly without any wispy stray hairs. Your make-up should be subtle and not caked on! Nails should be natural, short and without nail varnish, unless you are applying for a job as a nail technician. All jewellery including your watch should be removed.

There really is no excuse for a sloppy appearance. If you fail to do any of the above, you simply will not be offered the job.

From a professional point of view, there are a few things you must do during a trade test. It's easy to forget the simplest tasks when you are nervous, so familiarise yourself with the treatment basics:

- Prepare your work area with all the cotton wool, tissues, towels, products and equipment that you will need, including a disinfectant solution for sanitising tools and a record card.

Being asked what your weaknesses are is always a difficult question to answer because you can easily land yourself in it. Prepare an answer beforehand.

- Meet and greet the client with a big smile and friendly approach.
- Introduce yourself!
- Make a quick check of her medical history to ensure that she is suitable for treatment (even if she is a member of staff in the salon) and enter it onto a record card.
- Prepare her by giving her a gown and showing her to the couch or chair – help her onto the couch.
- If a gown is not available or suitable for the treatment, protect her clothing with a towel and couch roll.
- Ask her if she is comfortable and warm.
- Explain that you are going to wash your hands before you start.
- Explain what you are about to do before starting the treatment.
- Carry out the treatment with care and attention to detail.
- Check occasionally with the client that she is still comfortable.
- Keep your work area tidy throughout the treatment by throwing away waste immediately in a bin next to the work area and by replacing bottle tops straight away.
- Don't use your couch as a trolley top; this only shows bad habits and could result in spillage or accidents.
- When you have finished, help the client off the couch, ask her how she enjoyed it and, most importantly, thank her for her time.
- Wash your hands and return to your assessor for feedback.
- Hope for the best!

## TELEPHONE INTERVIEWS

Interviews by phone are becoming more popular with some employers in the hair and beauty industries. They are used as a first interview and can save valuable time for the company. If the employer likes the sound of you on the telephone, then you will be asked to attend a face-to-face interview. As with all interviews, preparation and organisation is the key. Don't ever get casual in your approach to job hunting.

You won't remember everything, so have your CV, application form, cover letter and the job application out in front of you before the call. It's a good idea to stand up when you are speaking; surprisingly enough, you will sound more businesslike and less casual than if you are slouching on a chair. Try to sound cheerful, enthusiastic and interested, and avoid using slang such as 'OK', 'yeah' or 'right'. For more advice about telephone interviews, see *Winning Interviews for First-time Job Hunters*.

## THE JOB OFFER

If you get to the interview stage but are unsuccessful, most companies are quite happy to give you feedback as to why you were not selected. This is helpful when applying for your next position. Learn by your experiences!

If, on the other hand, the company decides that you are the best person for the job, they will offer you the job – having first checked your references, of course. They may telephone you first and, if you accept, they will send you a formal letter outlining the offer. This will detail the terms and conditions – for example, what you will be paid, your hours of work, your holiday entitlement and so on. You need to check these out carefully before writing a formal letter of acceptance. Talk to the appropriate person on the telephone if you need anything clarified.

If you are not entirely satisfied with the terms and conditions of the job offer you may be in a position to negotiate, especially if you have a wealth of experience and technical skills (a newly qualified therapist, though, is not really in a position to negotiate). If this is the case, write a letter thanking the company for the offer of a job, explain that you are very keen to work with them but would like to know whether their formal offer terms are negotiable. Whatever aspect – pay, hours, holiday and so on – you would like improved upon, state this in the letter. Also explain that you will contact them within a day or two with a follow-up telephone call to discuss this further. They will then be in no doubt that you are still keen on the job.

*Negotiating a better deal can be risky and could cost you the job that you would have taken anyway.*

When you finally accept a job, you and the company will enter a contract of employment, which details the terms and conditions you have agreed upon. It is a legal requirement for employers to give you this in writing within two months of starting work for them.

Quite often the job will be offered on a trial period for a few months to check that you are suitable for the job. After this probationary time, if you have proved yourself, the job will become permanent.

Of course, you may decide to turn down the offer. Again, politeness and manners are the key – never alienate an employer as you may come across them later on in your career.

In the next chapter, we'll look more closely at the issue of pay. It can be a thorny issue in the beauty industry, and you need to be aware of your rights.

# Pay and perks

Traditionally, people working in the beauty industry were very poorly paid – something that helps explain the massive shortage of qualified workers today. However, things are changing and while starting salaries may still seem low, there are plenty of opportunities for much bigger salaries in the industry. Some typical annual incomes might be:

- for a newly qualified beauty therapist or nail technician – £8,000
- for an experienced beauty therapist – £10,000–£15,000
- for a salon or spa manager or owner – £15,000–£20,000.

There are likely to be regional variations in salaries for some positions. For example, working in a Central London salon, possibly with high-profile clients, you could earn substantially more than the figures indicated above. Salaries can also include an addition to the basic pay called London weighting, awarded because the cost of living in London is so high. Other parts of the UK are expensive to live and work in too, so ideally a salary ought to make an allowance for this. However, only when you have reached a senior position can you expect to benefit from regionally enhanced pay. This is why many graduates tend to work locally at first in order to gain much needed experience rather than travel to other parts of the country.

Employees have some protection against poor salaries – the minimum wage, which became law on 1 April 1999. From 1 October 2003, this gave workers the following entitlements:

- staff over 22 to be paid at least £4.50 per hour
- staff aged 18–21 to be paid at least £3.80 per hour.

From 1 October 2004, this will change:

- staff over 22 to be paid at least £4.85 per hour
- staff aged 18–21 to be paid at least £4.10 per hour.

It is an offence for an employer to pay an employee less. However, if you are over 22 and an employer provides accredited training whilst employing you (with an awarding body such as VTCT, Edexcel, City & Guilds and so on), then they only have to pay £3.80 per hour for the first six months as long as the training takes place for at least 26 days in that period.

There are government-funded schemes which entitle staff over 18 to the minimum wage if employed by a company. These schemes include –

- New Deal for the young unemployed
- New Deal for those aged 25 and above
- Work-Based Learning for Adults.

If you are on an Apprenticeship or Advanced Apprenticeship scheme, you will not be entitled to the minimum wage until the age of 19. Or, if you are over the age of 26, you will not be entitled to the NMW until after 12 months as an apprentice. More information is available on the Department of Trade and Industry website – www.dti.gov.uk – and at www.connexions.gov.uk.

## PERKS OF THE JOB

A job in the beauty industry has always provided a bonus – the chance to be pampered yourself! After all, it's just as important that you look as well-groomed and relaxed as your

> *A job in the beauty industry has always provided a bonus – the chance to be pampered yourself!*

clients. If there is a gap in the appointments column and there are no other jobs to be done, then it is accepted practice that staff carry out treatments or practise new skills on each other – as long as it doesn't affect their work.

It would never be acceptable, however, to book staff treatments in an appointment column at the expense of a paying client. Each company will have their own policy on staff treatments, and it is important that you check this beforehand. It may be, for instance, that the company asks its staff to make a small contribution towards the products used in the treatment.

## DID YOU KNOW?

The average number of clients visiting a small salon per week is 125 and for a large salon 265.

Other incentives on offer in some companies include commission payments based on your sales and occasionally your sales and treatments. This is particularly likely to be the case if you are a productive therapist who brings in a good profit for them – they will want to keep you as an employee and not lose you to another company. Commission can typically be 10 per cent of your takings (or more in some parts of the UK or in retailing jobs), so this can certainly boost your weekly wage.

A further perk is the tips. This is a very common occurrence in beauty-therapy establishments when clients are pleased with the treatment and service they have received.

This begs the question, of course – what exactly does make for excellent service and a professional treatment in the beauty industry? You'll have picked up many of the main points already, but in the next chapter we'll look more closely at the special qualities that go into the making of a truly excellent beauty specialist or therapist.

# 5

# Tools of the trade

Academic skills are important, but what makes a good, as opposed to a merely competent, beauty therapist are a few special attributes and qualities, many of which can be summed up as **people skills** – the ability to interact with all types of people from all walks of life regardless of age, ethnicity, gender or personality.

## THE MUST-HAVES

Being able to **make clients feel at ease** helps make sure they will rebook. Awkward silences and stilted conversations can make people feel embarrassed and self-conscious, especially when the type of treatment being carried out is of a very personal nature.

Some people are 'naturals' – they find it easy to talk to clients and are easy to warm to. Others find it harder, but many of these qualities will come with practice and experience. The most important personality qualities are –

- **good communication skills** – you must be good at explaining treatments and how products work
- **a smart appearance and good hygiene**

## DID YOU KNOW?

A small salon retains a higher percentage of clients than a large one. Is this perhaps due to better – that is, more personal – customer care?

- **a friendly and welcoming manner** that puts clients at ease
- **patience and good listening skills**
- **a positive attitude** – you have to show confidence and belief in the treatments and products you are offering
- **a caring and respectful manner**
- **stamina and strength** – you will be on your feet all day and some treatments (for example massage) are very strenuous
- **strong hands**
- **an ability to show calmness** when everything around you seems manic – a hectic or panic-stricken reaction when it's busy or when things don't go quite to plan will do nothing to reassure your client
- **good health and a high level of fitness**
- **artistic flair** – for example for nail art and make-up
- **knowledge of anatomy, physiology and chemistry or at least an aptitude to learn**
- **commercial ability** – for example, being able to work to recommended timescales for profit and commission
- **an ability to sell and promote** products and treatments to clients.

One other big quality needed when working in a salon, big or small, is the **ability to work as a team** and get on with a wide range of colleagues. This doesn't mean that you need to be best friends with everyone, but what it does mean is

Beauty therapy is a caring profession, so make sure that your actions and thoughts towards others reflect this.

that you will be expected to give and take – to be civil, friendly and cooperative.

One other big quality needed when working in a salon, big or small, is the ability to work as a team and get on with a wide range of colleagues.

## THE 'DEFINITELY NOTS'

There are some things that you won't be able to do much about but which will make a career in beauty therapy a bad choice. These might include medical reasons such as a bad back or allergies to lots of cosmetic products.

Bad attitude is something you can do something about, although some people refuse to believe that they are the ones with the problem! If you can't be bothered to put yourself out and always give the best that you can, then start looking for an alternative career now. Beauty therapy is a caring profession, so make sure that your actions and thoughts towards others reflect this. A short temper and unhelpful attitude are the last things needed in a busy salon. Clients can be demanding – and rightly so. They are paying money to be pampered and to receive a high standard of treatment.

# 6

# Treatments of the trade

If you're reading this book, you are clearly interested in taking up a career in beauty therapy, but how much of an idea do you really have of what it's all about? You may have had a few treatments yourself as a client, or you may even have done a few treatments for friends or neighbours on a casual basis, but many people are still surprised at just how involved beauty treatment is. It's not just a case of applying make-up or waxing a person's legs!

As well as the close personal contact, you will also be expected to operate mechanical and electrical machines as part of a treatment, have extensive knowledge of the muscles and bones and learn the science behind the treatments. In the box on the next page, you'll find a brief explanation of the main beauty treatments available in the UK today.

Many of the treatments listed are complex – and very occasionally things can go wrong. This is why all beauty specialists and therapists must have insurance. Insurance is not just a safety net in case you cause injury or damage to a client or her belongings; it is also there to protect you as a therapist. Unfortunately in today's world, people are making insurance claims against companies far more frequently than ever before so it is essential that you have extensive cover and abide by the rules and guidelines of the insurance policy in order to remain covered.

### A–Z OF BEAUTY TREATMENTS

If you think you want to be a Beauty Therapist make sure you know what treatments you will be expected to carry out.

**Aromatherapy** – Essential oils extracted from plant and herb sources are used through massage to alleviate a wide variety of conditions, to relieve stress and induce relaxation.

**Electrical body treatments** – A range of electrical equipment is used to achieve better muscle and skin tone. Some treatments aid slimming and improve the appearance of cellulite.

**Electrical epilation** – The removal of unwanted hair through the application of a low-level electrical current. Eventually the treatment can permanently destroy the hair.

**Electrical face treatments** – A range of electrical equipment is used to achieve better muscle and skin tone as well as for deep cleansing and anti-wrinkle treatments.

**Eye treatments** – This could include: eyelash tinting to darken lashes, eyebrow shaping to enhance the shape of the brow and eyebrow tinting to darken pale or grey brows. False lashes can also be applied to increase the length and thickness of the lashes.

**Fake (self) tanning** – This is tanning the safe way. The therapist applies a temporary tanning lotion to your body to deepen your natural skin tone.

**Heat and bath treatments** – Hydrotherapy (water therapy) can be very effective in relieving stress, aches and pains and as a preheating treatment prior to massage. Spa treatments are spa, steam and sauna.

**Indian head massage** – Also known as *champissage*, this is an ancient technique which involves massaging and rubbing the head, neck and shoulders. It is used for stress relief.

**Lash perming** – This enhances the lashes by temporarily curling them.

**Make-up** – Products used to enhance the natural appearance of the skin and facial features. Make-up effects can be for day or evening; they can be corrective, dramatic, theatrical, photographic and so on.

**Manicures and pedicures** – This involves treatment on skin of the hands and feet, the nails and the surrounding cuticles. Products are used to massage, remove dead dry skin, soften, shape and polish.

**Manual body massage** – Usually Swedish massage. Movements are used to improve the blood flow, exercise the muscles and relax the body. Hands are used for flowing movements such as stroking, friction movements such as kneading and stimulating movements such as beating and cupping.

**Manual facial** – This treatment deep-cleans the skin, exfoliates dead skin cells and removes blackheads; it also includes a massage of the face, neck and shoulders and a face mask. No electrical equipment is used, it is all hands-on.

**Nail techniques** – This involves applying extensions to the natural nail with gel or acrylic; it also includes nail art.

**Reflexology** – This consists of pressure massage on the reflex points of the hands or feet. These reflex points mirror the body. The treatment unblocks the energy lines to aid self-healing and body rebalancing.

**Ultraviolet (UV) tanning** – This is tanning of the skin by application of UV rays from a sunbed or solarium. This must be closely monitored by experienced staff so as not to permanently damage the skin.

**Wax depilation** – This is the removal of unwanted hair, usually on the legs, underarm, bikini and facial area. *Warm wax* is thinly applied to the skin. The wax sticks to the hairs, which enables them and their follicles to be removed when a paper or fabric strip is applied and pulled off again. *Hot wax* is applied thickly with a spatula and flicked off with the fingers.

With the increase in more specialised treatments such as laser, semi-permanent make-up and electrical treatments, there is more reason than ever to ensure good training that is industry recognised in order to get treatment liability cover.

It is essential that you have extensive insurance cover and abide by the rules and guidelines of the insurance policy in order to remain covered.

It takes a very long time to develop even a part of all the skills and knowledge needed in the beauty industry. Good basic training is a must, of course – but no one in this business really ever stops learning. In the following chapter, we'll look at what training actually involves and how you can continue to train and learn throughout your career.

# Training day

As we have already seen, training plays a crucial role in the beauty industry. In this chapter, we will look a little more carefully at each stage of the training process – from initial training at entry level into the professional to ongoing career development.

There is a wide range of courses and qualifications in the UK. It depends on different factors as to which method of training you choose – if you learn best by being continually assessed, then an NVQ/SVQ might be your best option; if you prefer to sit final examinations, then there are courses that offer this. We'll cover both these options below.

Training at private centres is usually shorter and more intensive than in further education colleges and with smaller class sizes. Private centres may not be approved to offer nationally recognised qualifications and have their own certificates of achievement. Take care – these are not always recognised as a valid qualification by employers. You must check what qualification you will get at the end of the private course because it may also be difficult to get insurance (see Chapter 6 for more on insurance).

## THE NVQ/SVQ ROUTE

The Hairdressing and Beauty Industry Authority (HABIA) states that there are no recommended formal entry requirements for acceptance into training for NVQ/SVQ Levels 1 and 2 and that the industry is more attracted by the qualities that a trainee has to offer. So, although some

NVQ1 → **BEAUTY THERAPY OR RECEPTION ASSISTANT**

SALONS, SPAS, HEALTH CLUBS

NVQ2 → **BEAUTY SPECIALIST**

CHOICE OF GENERAL, MAKE-UP OR NAIL SERVICES ROUTE

SALONS, MOBILE, NAIL BARS
OR RENT-A-CHAIR, COSMETIC COUNTERS

NVQ3 → **BEAUTY THERAPIST**

CHOICE OF GENERAL, MAKE-UP, NAIL SERVICES
OR SPA THERAPY ROUTE

SALONS, SPAS, SALON OWNER, THEATRE, TELEVISION,
HOSPITALS, COMPLEMENTARY THERAPY CENTRES,
ELECTROYSIS CLINICS, HEALTH CLUBS,
HEALTH FARMS, TRAINING CENTRES

Additional help in the form of learning support is available in further education colleges, so if you struggle with paperwork, can't get organised or have difficulty understanding some of the terminology or assignments, accept the help on offer in order to pass your course.

colleges do ask for GCSEs in Maths and English as a minimum entry requirement, learners are often judged on their individual merits even if they have not reached the required academic level to be accepted on a course.

NVQ/SVQs are made up of units and have a structure a little like building-blocks that build up to a complete qualification. There are strict criteria that a student must meet at every unit and every level in order for him or her to be judged competent at a particular skill. There are mandatory and optional units. Mandatory units cover the essential areas of the job and must be taken to pass the whole qualification, whereas optional units can be chosen to suit the student's own needs and preferences.

NVQs are work-related, competence-based qualifications. Completion of an NVQ shows that you can actually do the job and not just talk about it! NVQs reflect the skills and expertise needed to do a job well.

Standards are developed by Standards Setting Bodies or National Training Organisations (NTO's). The standards in Hairdressing and Beauty Therapy are set by HABIA.

These standards are mainly employer and industry led. In other words, employers tell the setting bodies:

- what they expect trainees to be learning in order to be successful in a job
- what they need to know and the skills they need to be able to demonstrate
- what they expect from their employees once in the salon.

Assessment for NVQ/SVQs is continuous throughout training and therefore avoids the need for a final examination. Assessment is carried out using various methods, including practical observation, written tasks and assignments and case studies. You'll also be expected to:

- compile a portfolio of evidence
- practise all skills on fellow students
- carry out practical treatments on clients
- sit end-of-unit tests.

Each practical skill must be assessed as competent in a **realistic working environment** and on a 'real client' in order for the student to be awarded that skill.

There is no set time limit for completion of an NVQ/SVQ, but after you have enrolled on a course you will be registered with the college and an awarding body. This registration will usually last up to three years, but if you take longer you will need to re-register and pay an additional fee along with extra tuition fees if requested by the college or centre. At a college of further education the average length of training on a full-time basis is one year for Level 2 and two years for Level 3.

At present there is not a complete NVQ/SVQ Level 4 structure for Beauty Therapy as it has been temporarily withdrawn and is undergoing development. Individual units of Level 4 may be available as an addition to the Level 3 qualifications in the near future, even if a complete award is not available. Level 4 units generally include organising staff in work and training, maintaining the financial side, business planning and keeping everything running smoothly – from the stock to the appointments!

## THE EXAMINATION ROUTE

Awarding bodies that offer the examination route are CIBTAC/CIDESCO and ITEC. If you follow this route, you will be expected to study for a set amount of hours laid down by the

---

**FOUNDATION APPRENTICESHIPS (FMAs in Wales or Skillseekers in Scotland) AND ADVANCED APPRENTICESHIPS (AMAs in Wales or MA in Scotland)**
This scheme is aimed at training and developing skills for 16 to 24-year-olds. It is a government initiative to train the potential high-fliers in Level 3 Beauty Therapy. The training is work-based so it provides an excellent opportunity for work experience as well as study. It has not proved as successful in Beauty Therapy as it has for Hairdressing as yet, but HABIA are aiming to resolve this for September 2004, believing that particularly the nails services and spa side of FA and AA training could be delivered quite well within the working environment.

To find out more, contact your local Learning and Skills Council (LSC) or Careers Office.

awarding body. At the end of the course, every student must sit a theory examination as well as a practical examination for each subject learnt. Check out the CIBTAC/CIDESCO and ITEC websites for more information about the content of both courses and what you need to do to pass.

Whilst ITEC subjects can be studied for at colleges of further education, CIDESCO and CIBTAC tend to be offered at private training establishments and as such can be expensive.

Once you've got that NVQ/SVQ or you've passed that ITEC exam, it's no good resting on your laurels. The beauty industry is a fast-moving sector and you need to keep as up to date as possible.

## FURTHER TRAINING AND CONTINUING PROFESSIONAL DEVELOPMENT (CPD)

Although there are some excellent basic qualification courses available out there, no one can learn everything at college. Once you've achieved your Beauty Therapy qualification you will need to continue your learning. A lot, of course, can be learnt through experience and years in practice, but additional and ongoing training will help to refresh, deepen and extend a therapist's knowledge and understanding. You may also want to train further in order to specialise.

This is especially true in industries like hairdressing and beauty therapy, where new techniques, products and equipment mean constant updating is essential for consistent and improving standards. Beauty therapy is a rapidly changing industry – practitioners need to keep up to date with the latest techniques and information and to continue the process of 'life-long learning'.

Indeed, ongoing training may eventually become compulsory for all beauty and holistic therapists. Until recently the abbreviation CPD – Continuing Professional Development – was familiar only to therapists working in education and nursing, where normally a certain number of hours of ongoing learning are required in order to keep your job. But this is no longer the case. Although CPD is currently only mandatory for assessors and verifiers of courses, it is considered good practice for everyone to develop and increase their skills on a regular basis.

If beauty and complementary therapy is finally regulated, it is likely that everyone will need to show evidence of continuing learning. There is no reason for anyone to wait until this becomes compulsory.  Start now and be ahead of the game. Here are a few tips to help you.

*Attendance at trade events, seminars and workshops will also count toward your Continuing Professional Development hours.*

- Spend every possible moment to develop your knowledge and practise your skills. Don't relax just because you have a qualification. Read every book, magazine and trade journal (see the lists in Chapter 9 – 'Resources') you can lay your hands on to get the latest beauty buzzword on everyone's lips. Clients expect you to know about what they might have read in an article – they look to you as the expert in the field of beauty.

- Attend trade shows and exhibitions (see Chapter 9) and workshops for professional development; never think you know it all just because you have qualified – you don't. Join professional organisations (see Chapter 9) to keep you informed about new developments and in contact with other therapists with whom you can share knowledge and advice.
- CPD in the industry is good practice. It will set you apart from the complacent comfortable existence of those who sit back and expect jobs and business to fall into their laps!
- Enrol on your next course now! Map out a five-year learning plan to extend your talents and flair and get a head start.

# The last word

# 8

Your head is now crammed with information and training options for Beauty Therapy. This book should have given you an insight into the industry so that now you can choose the career path that's right for you whether you are a new trainee or graduate. You now need to make the plunge – making the major decisions that will get you on the road to qualifications… and success!

The future looks bright if you:

- train in the basics first – there are no short cuts if you want your appointment columns full
- listen to your educators (that is, your college lecturers, trainers, assessors and employers) – together they have years of experience and will be ready with a wise word every now and then
- hear what people have to say and learn from them; don't get set in your ways – the industry develops and moves forward rapidly
- develop new skills and ideas continually
- teach others 'good practice' by example
- always strive to be the best you can.

Finally, good luck!

## THE LAST WORD

DO YOU LIKE WORKING WITH YOUR HANDS?

☐ YES
☐ NO

DO YOU LIKE WORKING CLOSELY WITH OTHER PEOPLE?

☐ YES
☐ NO

DO YOU CONSIDER YOURSELF TO BE FIT AND HEALTHY WITH GOOD STAMINA?

☐ YES
☐ NO

ARE YOU SELF MOTIVATED AND ABLE TO THINK ON YOUR FEET?

☐ YES
☐ NO

DO YOU WANT TO DO A JOB THAT MAKES PEOPLE FEEL GOOD ABOUT THEMSELVES?

☐ YES
☐ NO

DO YOU WANT TO SEE THE WORLD?

☐ YES
☐ NO

ARE YOU MOTIVATED TO LEARN NEW SKILLS?

☐ YES
☐ NO

If you answered 'YES' to all these questions then
CONGRATULATIONS! YOU'VE CHOSEN THE RIGHT CAREER!
If you answered 'NO' to any of these questions then this may not be the career for you.
However, you may like to consider some of the other careers detailed in the
'Real Life Guides' or 'Careers 2005' published by Trotman

# Resources

In this chapter you will find contact information for the relevant government and industry advisory, training, awarding and professional bodies for the beauty industry as well as further sources of information in the way of books, trade journals and websites. There is a wealth of information and advice out there – explore!

## AWARDING BODIES

These are the organisations that provide recognised qualifications within the beauty industry.

### City & Guilds

1 Giltspur Street
London
EC1A 9DD
020 7294 2800
www.city-and-guilds.co.uk

### Comité International d'Estéthique et de Cosmétologie (CIDESCO)

The Secretariat
Witikonerstrasse 365
8053 Zürich
Switzerland
00 41 1380 00 75
www.cidesco.com

**Confederation of International Beauty Therapy and Cosmetology (CIBTAC)**
Babtac House
70 Eastgate Street
Gloucester
GL1 1QN
01425 421114
www.cibtac.com

**Edexcel**
Stewart House
32 Russell Square
London
WC1B 5DN
0870 240 9800
www.edexcel.org.uk

**International Therapy Examinational Council (ITEC)**
4 Heathfield Terrace
Chiswick
London
W4 4JE
020 8994 4141
www.itecworld.co.uk

**Vocational Training and Charitable Trust  (VTCT)**
3rd Floor
Eastleigh House
Upper Market Street
Eastleigh
Hampshire
SO50 9FD
www.vtct.org.uk

## QUALIFICATION REGULATORY BODIES

### Hairdressing and Beauty Industry Authority (HABIA)
Fraser House
Nether Hall Road
Doncaster
DN1 2PH
01302 380013
www.habia.org

### Qualifications and Curriculum Authority (QCA)
83 Piccadilly
London
W1J 8QA
020 7509 5555
www.qca.org.uk

### Scottish Qualifications Authority (SQA)
Cadogan Suite, Hanover House
24 Douglas Street
Glasgow
G2 7NQ
0141 242 2332.
www.sqa.org.uk

## PROFESSIONAL MEMBERSHIP BODIES

### Association of Nail Technicians
Alexander House
Forehill
Ely
Cambridgeshire CB7 4ZA
01353 665577

**BABTAC**
British Association of Beauty Therapy and Cosmetology
Meteor Court
Barnett Way
Barnwood
Gloucester GL4 3GG
www.babtac.com

**British Association of Electrolysists**
sec@baeltd.fsbusiness.co.uk
www.electrolysis-bae-ltd.co.uk
0870 128 0477

**British Federation of Massage Practitioners**
www.jolanta.co.uk

**FHT**
Federation of Holistic Therapists
info@fht.org.uk
www.fht.org.uk
0870 420 2022

The FHT is made up of five special interest groups:

IFHB  – International Federation of Health & Beauty
        Therapists
ICHT  – International Council of Holistic Therapists
PACT – Professional Association of Clinical Therapists
HFST – International Council of Health, Fitness & Sports
        Therapists
ATL    – Association of Therapy Lecturers
HBEF – Health & Beauty Employers Federation

**Freelance Hair and Beauty Federation**
sabrahams@fhbf.org.uk
www.fhbf.org.uk

**The Guild**
Guild House
FREEPOST DY517
PO BOX 310
Derby DE23 9BR
info@beautyguild.com
www.beautyguild.com
0870 000 4242

**Institute of Electrolysis**
www.electrolysis.co.uk
0870 051 3611

**ITEC Professionals**
www.itecworld.co.uk
020 8994 4141

**Skillset**
The Sector Skills Council for the Audio Visual Industries
skillset.org or www.skillsformedia.com for the careers site.

## TRADE JOURNALS
The trade journals listed below are written exclusively for
everyone involved in the health and beauty industry and are
an authoritative source of professional information. The
journals are essential reading for keeping up to date with
treatment techniques, new products, cosmetic trends, trade
events and personalities influencing the trade. Editorial
coverage of news, technical articles and step-by-step

instructional features combine with advertisements for the latest equipment, products and treatments and jobs in the salon and spa to keep readers well informed. Contact their subscription departments using the listed contact details.

**Guild News**
11 issues per year
0870 000 4262

**Health and Beauty Salon**
12 issues per year
01444 445566

**International Therapist**
bi-monthly
only available to members of FHT
0870 420 2022

**Professional Beauty**
10 issues per year
01371 810433

**Professional Nails**
10 issues per year
01371 810433

**Professional Spa**
6 issues per year
01371 810433

**Professional Tanning**
free every quarter with *Professional Beauty*
01371 810433

**Salon Plus**
01353 665577

**Salon Today**
quarterly issues
020 8882 6064

**Scratch**
12 issues per year
www.creativenailplace.com
0845 225 2825

**Tanning World**
6 issues per year
www.beautyserve.co.uk

**Today's Therapist**
bi-monthly
0870 742 5069

**Vitality**
bi-monthly
available to members of BABTAC

**Warpaint**
6 issues per year
info@warpaint-makeup.com
01371 810433

# BOOKS

## BEAUTY THERAPY:

*Aesthetics for the Therapist: Theory and Practice*, Ann Hagman

*Anatomy and Physiology – Beauty Therapy Basics*, Helen McGuinness

*Beauty Therapy – The Basics (Level 2)*, Maxine Whittaker

*Beauty Therapy Fact File* (2nd edition), Janet Simms, Debbie Forsythe-Conroy and Judith Ifould

*Beauty Therapy: The Foundations – NVQ/SVQ Level 2*, Lorraine Nordman

*Body Therapy and Facial Work* (2nd edition), Mo Rosser

*The Beauty Salon and Its Equipment*, John V. Simmons

*Health and Beauty Therapy: A Practical Approach for NVQ Level 3*, D. Mernagh and J. Cartwright

*A Practical Guide to Beauty Therapy for NVQ Level 2* (2nd edition), Janet Simms

*S/NVQ Level 1: Introducing Beauty Therapy*, Samantha Taylor

*S/NVQ Level 2: Beauty Therapy*, Jane Hiscock and Frances Lovett

## ELECTROLYSIS:

*The Complete Guide to Electro-epilation*, Angela Wheat

*Electro-epilation – A Practical Approach*, Gill Morris, Elizabeth Cartwright and Michelle Severn

*Principles and Techniques for the Electrologist*, Ann Gallant

## SKIN AND MAKE-UP:

*Clinical Cosmetology*, Victoria L. Rayner

*The Complete Make-up Artist – Working in Film, Television and Theatre*, Penny Delamar

*Cosmetic Make-up and Manicure*, Ann Eaton and Florence Openshaw

*Skin Camouflage: A Guide to Remedial Techniques*, Joyce Allsworth

*Skin Care Beyond the Basics* (2nd edition), Mark Lees

*Stage Make-up*, Richard Corson

*The World of Skin Care*, Dr John Gray

**MASSAGE:**

*Baby Massage*, Helen McGuinness

*Body Massage for the Beauty Therapist*, Audrey Goldberg and Lucy McDonald

*Body Massage – Therapy Basics*, Mo Rosser

*The Complete Guide to Sports Massage*, Tim Paine

*Massage and Aromatherapy – A Practical Approach for NVQ Level 3* (2nd edition), Lyn Goldberg

*The Official Guide to Body Massage*, Adele O'Keefe

## BEAUTY PORTALS

### www.beautyawarenessweek.com

The BABTAC annual promotion – this promotion is aimed at introducing beauty therapy to people that might not have tried it before.

### www.thebeautybusiness.com

The consumer-driven beauty resource designed with the beauty professional in mind.

### www.beauty4students.co.uk

Excellent information and resource site for students, including monthly treatment features.

### www.beautymagonline.com

As online beauty magazines go, they don't come any better.

**www.beautyserve.com**
The Internet's most comprehensive beauty resource.

**www.connect2beauty.com**
An online beauty training company offering fully accredited NVQs.

## EXHIBITIONS

Exhibitions give companies in the industry the chance to promote their new treatments, products and equipment. They are also the ideal opportunity for Beauty and Holistic Therapists and Nail Technicians to see first-hand what's going on and to keep abreast of new developments. Visit www.professionalbeauty.co.uk and www.salonexhibitions.co.uk to find information on past and future exhibitions, including dates.

Important exhibitions include:

The London International Spa Convention
Professional Beauty Autumn
Professional Beauty Dublin
Professional Beauty
Professional Beauty North
Professional Nails
Salon International
Salon Scotland
Salon Spring
Warpaint

## COMPETITIONS

These give professionals the chance to show what they're made of, get free publicity and become a recognised name in the industry.

**British Beauty Awards**
Organised by *Health and Beauty Salon* magazine.

**Professional Beauty Consumer Awards**
**Professional Beauty Industry Awards**
Both these are organised by *Professional Beauty*,
*Professional Nails* and *Professional Spa* magazines.

## HEALTH AND BEAUTY RECRUITMENT SPECIALISTS

### Active Connection
Active Connection Limited
Epirus Mansions
3 Epirus Road
London
SW6 7UJ
020 7385 2388
www.activeconnection.co.uk

### Beauty Jobs Online
01372 363515
www.beautyjobsonline

### Red
1 Farnham Road
Guildford
GU2 4RG
01483 549022
www.redhotcareers.co.uk

**Spa Staff**
43 Mount Park Road
London
W5 2RS
020 8997 6426
www.spastaff.com

**Leisure Jobs**
Cloisters House
8 Battersea Park Road
London
SW8 4BG
0870 728 8000
www.leisurejobs.com